SUZANNE BYRD

ADHD and Relationships: A Woman's Perspective

First edition

This book was professionally typeset on Reedsy.
Find out more at reedsy.com

Contents

1

Understanding ADHD and Its Impact on Relationships

For women with ADHD, relationships can be uniquely challenging and rewarding. ADHD brings traits that can impact communication, task management, and emotional connection. But rather than viewing ADHD as a barrier, seeing it as a different way of processing the world can help both partners cultivate empathy, patience, and understanding. By recognizing ADHD traits and their impact on relationships, women can work with their partners to create a foundation of trust and mutual support.

ADHD manifests differently in women compared to men. Many women experience a range of traits—such as impulsivity, distractibility, emotional sensitivity, and hyper-focus—each affecting relationship dynamics. Understanding how these characteristics impact romantic relationships can help women and their partners better navigate potential conflicts and find ways to connect that honor both partners' needs.

Recognizing Common ADHD Traits in Relationships

1. Impulsivity and Reactivity

Women with ADHD may react impulsively in conversations or decisions. They might say something without thinking, interrupt, or change topics quickly, which can sometimes leave a partner feeling unheard or sidelined. Impulsivity can also manifest in behaviors like making spontaneous plans, which might feel exhilarating for one partner but destabilizing for the other.

2. Distractibility and Forgetfulness

ADHD often impacts attention and memory. Women with ADHD might struggle to stay focused during conversations or forget important details about their partner's day. This trait can sometimes be misinterpreted as a lack of interest or care, even when it's unintentional.

3. Hyper-Focus on Specific Interests

Hyper-focus is a common ADHD trait where individuals become so engrossed in a task that they lose track of time and ignore other responsibilities. This can lead to misunderstandings, as partners may feel neglected when the individual with ADHD is deeply focused on work or a hobby.

4. Emotional Sensitivity and Intensity

Many women with ADHD experience emotions intensely and are highly sensitive to their partner's moods. This can lead to strong emotional reactions or feeling overwhelmed during disagreements. Emotional sensitivity can be both a challenge and a strength, as women with ADHD are often empathetic and emotionally attuned to their partners.

5. Difficulty with Organization and Time Management

Managing schedules, planning dates, or dividing household responsibilities can be difficult for women with ADHD. Forgetting appointments, struggling to keep up with routines, or misplacing important items may inadvertently frustrate partners.

Understanding these ADHD traits and how they manifest in relationships allows women and their partners to approach challenges constructively rather than with frustration or resentment.

Case Study: Sarah's Journey of Self-Awareness and Relationship Growth

Sarah, a 34-year-old with ADHD, had always felt that her marriage was strained because of her behaviors. Her husband, Dave, didn't understand why she was so forgetful or why their conversations sometimes felt disjointed. They often argued, particularly about household responsibilities and communication breakdowns.

After being diagnosed with ADHD, Sarah realized that many of her behaviors were influenced by her condition rather than personal flaws. Her forgetfulness and impulsivity were not signs of irresponsibility but symptoms of ADHD. This shift in perspective led Sarah to initiate an open conversation with Dave about how ADHD shaped her experiences.

Sarah's Steps to Foster Understanding in Her Relationship

1. Educating Her Partner

Sarah shared resources with Dave about ADHD, helping him understand how it impacted her day-to-day interactions. Dave read articles and joined her in watching videos about ADHD in relationships, which allowed him to empathize and better grasp the challenges Sarah faced.

2. Collaborating on Solutions to Support Each Other

Together, they created a weekly "household meeting" where they discussed responsibilities for the week, checked in on each other's needs, and planned out shared tasks. By dividing responsibilities and adjusting expectations, both partners felt more supported.

Through these conversations, Sarah and Dave developed a deeper understanding of each other, turning ADHD-related challenges into opportunities for growth.

Practical Strategies for Women with ADHD to Foster Understanding in Relationships

1. Reflect on Your ADHD Traits

Take time to explore how ADHD influences your behavior in relationships. Journaling about specific ADHD traits (e.g., impulsivity, emotional intensity) and observing how they impact interactions with your partner can offer clarity and self-awareness. Understanding these traits can help you express them to your partner, allowing for more constructive conversations.

2. Embrace ADHD as Part of Your Identity

Accepting ADHD as a part of yourself rather than something to "fix" can shift the relationship dynamic. This mindset encourages your partner to approach ADHD with curiosity and empathy, understanding that these traits are integral to who you are.

3. Initiate an Honest Conversation with Your Partner

Openly share how ADHD impacts your daily experiences and ask your partner about their perspective. Aim to communicate specific behaviors or challenges you'd like support with, as well as areas where you feel confident. This honest exchange can foster mutual understanding and set the stage for collaborative problem-solving.

4. Establish Supportive Routines Together

Many couples find that implementing routines helps balance the relationship dynamic. For example, scheduling a weekly planning session for household chores or setting aside designated times for quality time can reduce misunderstandings and provide structure. Using tools like shared calendars or whiteboards can also help both partners stay aligned.

5. Recognize and Celebrate ADHD Strengths

ADHD often brings unique strengths, such as creativity, empathy, and spontaneity, which can enrich relationships. Reflect on the positive aspects of ADHD and consider how they contribute to your partnership. Celebrating these strengths together can help reframe ADHD as an asset rather than a burden.

Practical Exercise: Creating a Relationship "User Guide"

One practical tool to foster understanding is to create a "user guide" about yourself. This guide can outline your ADHD-related needs, preferences, and strengths. Here's how to create one:

1. Identify Key Traits: List specific ADHD traits that impact your relationship, such as "I tend to forget dates unless they're written down" or "I get emotionally overwhelmed during arguments."

2. Explain Your Needs: For each trait, describe ways your partner can support you. For instance, "If I forget a task, a gentle reminder helps more than a confrontation."

3. Highlight Strengths: Include ADHD-related strengths you bring to the relationship, like "I am very empathetic" or "I am open to spontaneous plans."

4. Review Together: Share the guide with your partner as a conversation starter, allowing both of you to discuss and adapt to each other's needs.

Sarah and Dave found that developing a "user guide" for each other provided valuable insights into how to support each other better. By understanding each other's challenges and strengths, they could approach their relationship with greater compassion.

Embracing ADHD as a Foundation for Growth

Recognizing the impact of ADHD on relationships allows women to view their traits with understanding rather than shame. Embracing these traits and communicating them openly to a partner fosters an environment where both individuals feel supported and respected. By focusing on ADHD not as a limitation but as a unique perspective, women with ADHD can create strong, fulfilling partnerships that thrive on mutual empathy and collaboration.

2

Self-Acceptance as the Foundation of Healthy Relationships

Self-acceptance is essential for creating a healthy and fulfilling relationship, especially for women with ADHD. When you accept ADHD as a part of who you are, you can navigate relationships with authenticity and confidence, setting realistic expectations for yourself and your partner. Self-acceptance reduces the need to hide or mask ADHD traits, which can lead to burnout, resentment, or a sense of inadequacy.

In many cases, women with ADHD have spent years trying to "fit in" or appear neurotypical, often at the expense of their well-being. Society often rewards behaviors like organization, timeliness, and emotional stability—traits that may be more challenging for individuals with ADHD. Accepting oneself as neurodivergent means recognizing these challenges as part of one's identity, not as personal flaws.

Maya's Journey: Embracing Self-Compassion

Maya, a 32-year-old with ADHD, struggled with perfectionism and self-doubt. In her relationships, she constantly feared that her ADHD would make her a burden. To avoid this, she would go to great lengths to keep up with her partner's expectations, trying to be punctual, organized, and emotionally steady—traits that didn't come naturally to her. However, this masking led her to feel exhausted, frustrated, and guilty whenever she fell short.

When Maya received her ADHD diagnosis, she experienced a profound shift in perspective. She began to see her ADHD as a part of her identity rather than something to hide or fix. This mindset shift opened the door to self-compassion and allowed her to be more honest with herself and her partner about her needs.

Steps Maya Took to Cultivate Self-Acceptance:

1. Reframing ADHD as a Neurodivergence, Not a Weakness

Maya educated herself on ADHD and embraced it as a different way of processing information rather than a flaw. By understanding ADHD traits and how they influenced her, she reframed challenges like forgetfulness or impulsivity as simply part of her neurodivergent experience.

2. Setting Boundaries that Honor Her Needs

Maya stopped overcommitting herself to social events or responsibilities just to appear "normal." She began setting boundaries, saying "no" when necessary, and managing her energy wisely.

Setting boundaries helped her avoid burnout and allowed her to show up in her relationship authentically.

3. Practicing Self-Compassion in Daily Life

Maya started incorporating self-compassion exercises into her daily routine, such as taking breaks when she felt overwhelmed and speaking kindly to herself when she made mistakes. These small acts reinforced a positive relationship with herself, allowing her to treat her ADHD-related challenges with empathy.

Through these steps, Maya found a renewed sense of confidence. She communicated her needs to her partner, explaining that while she valued their relationship, she also needed space to manage her energy and honor her limits.

Practical Exercises for Cultivating Self-Acceptance

1. Self-Reflection Journaling

Dedicate a journal to exploring your ADHD traits and how they affect your life. Reflect on questions like, "What challenges do I face because of ADHD?" and "What strengths does ADHD bring to my relationships?" This journaling practice can help clarify which ADHD-related traits you want to embrace, allowing you to see them with more empathy.

2. Daily Self-Compassion Practice

Each day, take a few moments to practice self-compassion. This can be as simple as pausing when you feel frustrated and telling yourself, "It's okay to struggle sometimes." Small acts of self-compassion can build a habit of treating yourself kindly, helping you accept ADHD traits without guilt or shame.

3. Identify Personal ADHD Strengths

ADHD often brings unique strengths, such as creativity, empathy, and adaptability. Make a list of traits you appreciate about yourself, specifically those influenced by ADHD. Recognize how these strengths benefit your relationships, whether it's by adding spontaneity or making you a more empathetic listener.

4. Challenge Negative Self-Talk

Notice when you're being critical of yourself, particularly about ADHD-related behaviors. Instead of focusing on mistakes, try to reframe them as learning experiences. For example, if you forgot an appointment, acknowledge it without self-blame and consider how you might approach it differently next time.

Case Study: How Maya's Self-Acceptance Changed Her Relationship

Before her journey to self-acceptance, Maya often found herself apologizing to her partner for behaviors she couldn't control, like running late or feeling emotionally overwhelmed. Her partner didn't understand the depth of her struggle, which left Maya feeling isolated and ashamed.

After working on self-acceptance, Maya approached her partner with openness. She explained her ADHD traits and how they influenced her actions, making it clear that these traits weren't personal shortcomings but part of her neurodivergent experience. She also shared strategies she was using to manage these challenges, like setting reminders for herself or practicing self-compassion.

Her partner responded with empathy, appreciating Maya's honesty and learning more about how to support her. By embracing herself, Maya created a stronger foundation for her relationship. She stopped masking her ADHD, and her partner saw the real her, which strengthened their connection.

Practical Tips for Building Self-Acceptance in Relationships

1. Be Open About ADHD with Your Partner

Sharing your ADHD journey can help demystify your experiences for your partner, fostering empathy and understanding. Rather than framing ADHD traits as problems, present them as part of who you are and discuss ways your partner can support you.

2. Set Realistic Expectations and Honor Your Limits

Rather than striving to meet neurotypical expectations, set goals that honor your ADHD strengths and limitations. If certain activities or commitments are challenging, be honest about them, and create a plan with your partner that allows you to navigate these challenges in a balanced way.

3. Celebrate Small Wins Together

In moments when you achieve something despite ADHD challenges, celebrate it with your partner. Whether it's following through on a plan or completing a task on time, these small victories build self-confidence and show your partner how resilient you are.

4. Seek Out Stories of Women with ADHD

Reading about other women's ADHD journeys can provide validation and reduce feelings of isolation. Connecting with others who share similar challenges reinforces that ADHD is a common experience and reminds you that you're not alone in facing it.

Embracing ADHD in Relationships as a Source of Strength

Self-acceptance enables women with ADHD to approach relationships without the fear of being judged. When you accept your traits and communicate them honestly, you allow your partner to see the authentic you, creating room for genuine connection. Rather than masking or hiding, embracing ADHD lets you focus on what makes you unique, using it as a source of strength rather than a perceived flaw.

As Maya's story shows, self-acceptance is a journey. By recognizing ADHD as an integral part of your identity, you can foster a relationship that feels safe, supportive, and understanding. When women with ADHD choose self-compassion over self-criticism, they create a foundation of self-love that extends to their relationships, allowing them to connect with others authentically and confidently.

3

Communication Techniques that Work

Effective communication is the backbone of any healthy relationship, but for women with ADHD, certain communication challenges can arise. Impulsivity, distractibility, and a tendency to overthink can make it difficult to convey thoughts clearly, stay engaged in conversations, or avoid misunderstandings. Fortunately, with intentional techniques and practice, women with ADHD can develop communication skills that support meaningful, productive conversations with their partners.

For Ella, a 28-year-old with ADHD, communication had always been challenging. Her impulsivity often led her to interrupt her partner or speak without fully processing her thoughts. As a result, conversations sometimes escalated into conflicts, leaving her partner feeling unheard and Ella feeling frustrated. Over time, however, Ella learned to implement communication techniques that helped her respond rather than react, creating a more harmonious dynamic in her relationship.

The Role of ADHD in Communication Challenges

1. Impulsivity and Over-Talking

Many women with ADHD find themselves speaking impulsively, interrupting others, or jumping from one topic to another. This can sometimes overwhelm a partner or make them feel sidelined in conversations.

2. Difficulty Staying Focused

Distractibility can make it hard to stay engaged, especially during lengthy or complex conversations. Partners may feel that the woman with ADHD isn't fully present or invested in the discussion, even when this is unintentional.

3. Emotional Reactivity

ADHD can amplify emotional responses, causing individuals to react strongly during disagreements. Quick reactions can sometimes lead to misunderstandings or escalated conflicts, making it hard to resolve issues calmly.

4. Overthinking and Anxiety

Some women with ADHD may worry about how they're perceived in conversations, leading to self-consciousness or overthinking. This can make it difficult to engage openly, as they may second-guess their responses or avoid discussing certain topics.

Understanding how these traits impact communication is the

first step in developing techniques to address them. With the right strategies, women with ADHD can learn to manage impulsivity, stay engaged, and communicate with intention.

Practical Communication Techniques for Women with ADHD

1. Pause and Breathe Before Responding

Taking a brief pause before responding can help reduce impulsive reactions and allow time to organize thoughts. This pause can be as simple as taking a deep breath or mentally counting to three. Practicing this technique helps avoid interruptions and allows for more thoughtful responses.

Example: When Ella's partner brought up a concern about their budget, she felt an immediate urge to defend her spending habits. Instead of reacting impulsively, she took a deep breath, which gave her time to process her response calmly.

2. Use "I" Statements

Framing statements with "I feel" or "I think" helps keep conversations constructive and reduces defensiveness. For example, instead of saying, "You never listen to me," try, "I feel unheard when we're discussing certain topics." This approach shifts the focus to personal feelings, fostering empathy and reducing potential conflict.

Example: Ella practiced using "I" statements during challenging conversations, which helped her communicate her feelings without making her partner feel blamed or criticized.

3. Practice Active Listening

Active listening involves fully focusing on the speaker, maintaining eye contact, and showing interest through verbal or non-verbal cues like nodding. This helps prevent the mind from wandering and demonstrates engagement. If you find yourself drifting, gently redirect your focus back to the conversation without self-criticism.

Example: Ella found that maintaining eye contact helped her stay grounded in conversations, making her partner feel more valued and heard.

4. Clarify When Needed

Asking questions to confirm understanding can prevent miscommunications, especially during complex or emotionally charged conversations. Phrases like "Did I understand that correctly?" or "Can you clarify what you mean?" can clear up potential misunderstandings and ensure that both partners are on the same page.

Example: During a recent conversation about future goals,

Ella's partner used some ambiguous language. Instead of assuming, she asked for clarification, which helped them avoid a miscommunication.

5. Set Boundaries for High-Emotion Conversations

In moments of high emotion, it can be helpful to set boundaries around the conversation. For instance, agreeing to a "timeout" if emotions escalate can prevent either partner from saying something they might regret. If emotions start to rise, respectfully ask for a brief pause and commit to returning to the conversation once both partners have had time to cool down.

Example: Ella and her partner established a mutual agreement to take a five-minute break whenever conversations became too heated. This gave both of them time to reflect before continuing the discussion.

Case Study: Ella's Transformation from Reactive to Responsive

At the start of her relationship, Ella often felt like her communication style created a barrier between her and her partner. She would jump into conversations with strong opinions, often without fully listening to her partner's perspective. Over time, these impulsive reactions led to frustration on both sides, with her partner feeling unheard and Ella feeling misunderstood.

Realizing the impact of her communication style, Ella decided to incorporate specific strategies. She practiced the three-second rule, pausing to take a breath before responding. She also made an effort to use "I" statements and active listening techniques, which helped her stay present and avoid misunderstandings. These changes, though small, had a profound effect on her relationship.

Example Conversation Transformation:

Before: Ella's partner might say, "I'm feeling stressed about our financial goals." Ella, reacting impulsively, might respond, "You're always stressed about something."

After: With practice, Ella's new response became, "I hear that you're feeling stressed. Is there a specific part of our finances you're worried about?" This response showed empathy and opened the door for constructive conversation.

These simple shifts allowed Ella to communicate with greater intention, creating a more balanced and supportive dynamic with her partner. By replacing impulsivity with mindfulness, Ella's partner felt more understood, and their conversations became more productive.

Additional Tips for Partners Supporting Women with ADHD

Effective communication is a two-way street. Partners can help support their loved one's communication by fostering a safe, non-judgmental environment. Here are a few ways partners can provide support:

1. Provide Gentle Reminders Without Judgment

If your partner tends to interrupt or change topics, consider offering gentle reminders without sounding critical. For example, "I'd like to finish my thought first, and then I'd love to hear yours."

2. Encourage Breaks When Emotions Escalate

Agree on a mutual plan for timeouts during emotionally charged moments. If conversations start to feel overwhelming, either partner can request a break without guilt or shame.

3. Acknowledge Effort and Progress

Recognizing the effort it takes for your partner to adopt new communication techniques can be incredibly motivating. Simple acknowledgments like, "I appreciate how you listened without interrupting" can reinforce positive behavior and foster growth.

Embracing Communication as a Skill to Build Together

Effective communication doesn't come naturally to everyone, but it can be developed through practice and patience. For women with ADHD, learning these skills may require extra effort, but the rewards are worth it. As Ella's journey demonstrates, small changes in conversation style can lead to significant improvements in relationship satisfaction. By practicing mindfulness, using "I" statements, and taking time to pause, women with ADHD can foster deeper connections and reduce misunderstandings.

When partners work together to communicate effectively, they build a relationship that thrives on mutual understanding, empathy, and respect. Embracing communication as a skill, rather than a fixed trait, allows both partners to grow and adapt, creating a foundation for a strong, resilient connection.

4

Navigating Emotional Regulation in Intimate Relationships

Emotional regulation is one of the most challenging aspects of ADHD, particularly in intimate relationships. For many women with ADHD, emotions can feel intense and overwhelming, often leading to impulsive reactions or difficulties in managing strong feelings. Learning tools to regulate emotions effectively can empower women to handle conflicts and build stronger, more supportive relationships with their partners.

Emotional regulation doesn't mean suppressing emotions; instead, it's about developing strategies to understand, process, and express emotions in a healthy way. Women with ADHD can benefit greatly from learning grounding techniques, mindfulness practices, and ways to communicate their emotional needs. These skills foster a sense of balance and create an environment where both partners feel understood and respected.

Understanding ADHD and Emotional Intensity

1. Heightened Sensitivity to Criticism and Rejection

Many women with ADHD experience what is often called Rejection Sensitivity Dysphoria (RSD). This heightened sensitivity can make even small criticisms feel intense and personal, which can lead to quick defensive reactions or shutting down emotionally.

2. Difficulty with Emotional Self-Regulation

Managing emotions in the heat of the moment can be difficult. Women with ADHD might find that they go from calm to frustrated or anxious very quickly, especially during disagreements. This intensity can lead to saying things they don't mean or withdrawing from the conversation.

3. Emotional "Flooding" and Overwhelm

When emotions reach a certain intensity, it can feel like being "flooded" with feelings. At this point, rational thought can become difficult, and the focus shifts to managing the immediate emotional reaction rather than resolving the issue at hand.

4. Hyper-Responsiveness to Partner's Emotions

Women with ADHD are often highly empathetic, which can sometimes result in absorbing their partner's emotions. This can lead to feeling responsible for their partner's moods, which creates added emotional pressure.

Understanding these emotional patterns can help women with ADHD identify the triggers and responses that may affect their relationships. Learning emotional regulation skills enables them to manage these responses constructively, leading to healthier, more supportive dynamics.

Practical Techniques for Emotional Regulation

1. Mindfulness and Breathing Exercises

Mindfulness practices, such as deep breathing or body scans, help slow down the mind and body during moments of intense emotion. Focusing on deep breaths signals to the body to relax, which helps create space to process feelings before reacting. The "4-7-8" breathing technique—inhale for four counts, hold for seven, and exhale for eight—can be especially effective in calming the nervous system.

Example: During a heated conversation, Jenna found herself becoming anxious and defensive. She used the 4-7-8 breathing technique, which helped her regain a sense of calm and allowed her to continue the discussion without feeling overwhelmed.

2. Name the Emotion Out Loud

Verbally naming an emotion, like saying "I feel frustrated" or "I'm feeling anxious," helps create a slight distance from the feeling. By identifying the emotion, it becomes easier to process it without letting it take over. Naming the emotion also communicates to a partner what's going on internally, fostering understanding.

Example: Jenna noticed that simply saying, "I feel really frustrated right now," helped her partner understand her state of mind, which allowed him to respond with empathy rather than defensiveness.

3. Grounding Techniques for Moments of High Emotion

Grounding techniques help redirect attention to the present moment and the physical body, reducing feelings of emotional overwhelm. Examples include pressing feet firmly on the ground, holding a textured object, or focusing on physical sensations like the feel of fabric or the sound of nearby noises.

Example: When Jenna felt emotionally flooded, she practiced grounding by placing her hands on a cold glass of water, focusing on the temperature and texture. This sensory connection helped her stay present and reduced the intensity of her emotions.

4. Using a Timeout Strategy

During moments of heightened emotion, it can be beneficial to take a brief "timeout." By stepping away for a few minutes, women with ADHD can avoid reactive responses and allow themselves time to process emotions. Agreeing with a partner on a specific phrase like "Let's pause for a moment" creates a non-judgmental way to take a break.

Example: Jenna and her partner established a rule to take a five-minute timeout during intense arguments. This pause helped her gain perspective and continue the conversation with a clearer mind.

5. Create a "Feelings Journal" to Process Emotions

Keeping a journal to document feelings helps with emotional reflection and self-awareness. Writing down thoughts after an intense moment allows for more thorough processing and can provide insights into patterns and triggers. Reviewing this journal can help women with ADHD identify recurring emotions or challenges in their relationships.

Example: Jenna kept a small journal where she wrote about her emotional responses during conflicts. Over time, this helped her notice patterns, like feeling more reactive when she was stressed from work, allowing her to address these factors proactively.

Case Study: Jenna's Success with Mindfulness and Grounding Techniques

Jenna, a 35-year-old woman with ADHD, often found herself in arguments with her partner, Tom. Her emotions would escalate quickly, making it hard to think clearly. In the heat of the moment, Jenna would sometimes say things she didn't mean, leading to guilt and frustration. Her partner, feeling overwhelmed by Jenna's intensity, would often withdraw from the argument, leaving both of them feeling misunderstood.

Recognizing the impact of her emotional intensity on her relationship, Jenna decided to try a few techniques. She practiced grounding exercises, like focusing on deep breathing, which helped her stay calm during disagreements. Jenna also used a "feelings journal" to document her emotions after each argument, identifying common triggers and reflecting on ways to manage them.

Over time, Jenna noticed a positive shift. She felt more in control during conversations, and Tom appreciated her efforts to manage her reactions. By practicing mindfulness and grounding, Jenna created a more balanced approach to handling emotions, leading to a more harmonious dynamic with her partner.

Tips for Partners to Support Emotional Regulation

1. Encourage Open Communication About Emotions

Encourage your partner to share their feelings openly, without judgment or criticism. This creates a safe environment where they feel comfortable expressing emotions rather than suppressing them, which can prevent escalated reactions.

2. Remain Patient During Emotional Moments

Emotional regulation is a skill that requires practice. Offer patience and understanding if your partner is working to manage intense emotions, and avoid taking emotional reactions personally.

3. Validate Their Emotions

Acknowledging your partner's feelings, even if you don't fully understand them, can help them feel supported. Statements like "I can see that this is really hard for you" can provide reassurance and comfort, reducing feelings of defensiveness or isolation.

Embracing Emotional Growth in Relationships

Learning emotional regulation skills is an ongoing journey, especially for women with ADHD, who may experience heightened sensitivity and emotional intensity. By implementing mindfulness techniques, grounding exercises, and establishing safe spaces for emotional expression, women with ADHD can cultivate a balanced, self-aware approach to managing emotions. This not only enhances their well-being but also strengthens their relationships by reducing misunderstandings and creating an environment where both partners feel valued and supported.

Jenna's journey illustrates that emotional regulation is a skill that can be developed and refined. With practice, women with ADHD can foster a healthier relationship dynamic that respects and honors both partners' emotional needs. Emotional growth requires patience, self-compassion, and open communication, building a foundation for resilient, empathetic relationships.

5

Building Effective Routines and Shared Responsibilities

Managing household tasks, creating routines, and sharing responsibilities can be challenging for women with ADHD. With difficulties in organization, task initiation, and follow-through, it's easy for daily responsibilities to feel overwhelming, leading to frustration for both partners. However, building effective routines and collaboratively managing responsibilities can bring a sense of structure and balance to the home, reducing tension and fostering cooperation.

For Priya, a 29-year-old teacher with ADHD, household responsibilities often felt like an insurmountable burden. Her partner frequently expressed frustration when chores were left unfinished, leading Priya to feel guilty and defensive. Recognizing the strain this placed on their relationship, Priya and her partner worked together to create routines and shared systems that honored her unique needs. With patience, communication, and trial and error, they developed strategies that helped them maintain a harmonious home life.

Understanding ADHD Challenges with Routine and Task Management

1. Task Initiation and Follow-Through

Women with ADHD may struggle with initiating tasks, especially those that feel mundane or overwhelming. Even after starting a task, it can be difficult to maintain focus and see it through to completion, leading to unfinished chores and a sense of frustration.

2. Difficulty with Time Management

Time often feels abstract for those with ADHD, making it challenging to estimate how long tasks will take or allocate time effectively. This can lead to last-minute scrambles, missed commitments, or neglected responsibilities.

3. Sensory Overwhelm

Household tasks can sometimes feel overstimulating, especially chores involving strong smells, textures, or sounds. This sensory sensitivity can lead women with ADHD to avoid certain tasks, contributing to feelings of guilt or inadequacy.

4. Task Switching and Mental Exhaustion

Moving from one task to another, especially when switching between different types of activities, can be mentally exhausting. ADHD can make it challenging to transition smoothly, which can contribute to a sense of overwhelm or lead to procrastination.

By acknowledging these challenges and working with their partner to address them, women with ADHD can find ways to create routines and shared responsibilities that feel achievable and sustainable.

Practical Strategies for Building Effective Routines

1. Collaborate on a Weekly Planning Session

Designate a time each week to discuss responsibilities, set goals, and plan household tasks together. This provides clarity for both partners and reduces stress. During these sessions, outline priorities for the week and decide who will handle which tasks. Having a clear roadmap can make responsibilities feel more manageable.

Example: Priya and her partner set aside Sunday evenings as their "planning time," where they reviewed upcoming commitments, outlined household chores, and set shared goals for the week.

2. Use Visual Reminders and Checklists

Visual aids, like chore charts or whiteboards, help break tasks into manageable steps and provide a sense of accomplishment as items are completed. For women with ADHD, seeing tasks visually can reinforce memory and accountability. Consider using a shared calendar or a task management app to coordinate schedules and remind each other of important dates.

Example: Priya used a shared online calendar with her partner, which helped keep both of them accountable and reminded her of tasks without relying on memory alone.

3. Assign Tasks Based on Strengths and Preferences

Dividing tasks according to each partner's strengths and preferences can make household responsibilities feel less burdensome. For example, if one partner enjoys cooking, they might take on meal prep while the other handles grocery shopping. Working together to divide chores according to comfort and ability promotes balance and reduces stress.

Example: Priya found that her partner preferred cooking, while she enjoyed planning meals. By dividing these tasks accordingly, they created a more enjoyable and efficient routine.

4. Establish Routine "Reset" Days

Designate one day each week as a "reset day" for catching up on any tasks that were missed or left incomplete. This designated day allows for flexibility throughout the week, while still ensuring that responsibilities are addressed. For example, a "Saturday Reset" might include tidying the home, laundry, and preparing for the week ahead.

Example: Priya and her partner used Saturdays as their reset day, which helped them tackle lingering tasks and ensured their home felt organized for the upcoming week.

5. Break Down Large Tasks into Smaller Steps

Big tasks, like organizing a room or deep cleaning, can feel overwhelming, especially for those with ADHD. Breaking these tasks into smaller steps, such as focusing on one section at a time, can make them feel more manageable. Small, consistent steps reduce the pressure and build a sense of accomplishment.

Example: When tackling spring cleaning, Priya and her partner broke the job into smaller parts, like "organize the closet" or "dust the living room," rather than attempting the whole house at once.

Case Study: Priya and Her Partner's Journey to Collaborative Household Management

Before implementing these strategies, Priya's partner often felt that household chores were left unfinished or overlooked, which led to misunderstandings and frustration. Priya, on the other hand, felt overwhelmed by vague expectations and found it challenging to manage all her responsibilities without clear guidelines.

By introducing weekly planning sessions and using visual reminders, Priya and her partner found a new rhythm that worked for them. Her partner began to appreciate Priya's efforts and understand her ADHD challenges, while Priya felt more confident and capable. This collaborative approach allowed both partners to feel more supported and reduced the friction caused by household responsibilities.

Additional Tips for Managing Shared Responsibilities

1. Allow Flexibility When Needed

Life doesn't always go according to plan, so flexibility is essential. If a chore isn't completed on time, approach it with understanding rather than criticism. Adapting to unexpected changes allows for greater resilience and reduces stress for both partners.

2. Acknowledge Efforts and Celebrate Progress

each other's efforts, however small, builds morale and reinforces positive behavior. Offering a simple "thank you" or celebrating completed tasks fosters appreciation and creates a more supportive environment.

3. Set Realistic Expectations and Give Grace for Imperfection

Understand that routines are meant to provide structure, not to impose rigidity. If tasks aren't completed perfectly, remember that effort matters more than perfection. Approaching routines with flexibility helps prevent burnout and creates a more enjoyable household dynamic.

4. Make Tasks Enjoyable with Music or Rewards

Introducing small rewards or adding enjoyable elements to chores can make them more engaging. For example, playing music while cleaning or treating yourself to a coffee break after completing a task can add motivation and make chores feel less tedious.

Embracing Routines as Tools for Harmony, Not Rigidity

Effective routines don't have to be rigid or overwhelming. For women with ADHD, creating routines that honor their strengths, needs, and preferences can help make household responsibilities feel achievable and rewarding. When routines are developed collaboratively, they become tools for balance rather than sources of stress.

As Priya's journey shows, building routines and sharing responsibilities requires open communication, patience, and flexibility. By planning together, using visual aids, and setting realistic expectations, women with ADHD and their partners can foster a harmonious home environment. Shared routines encourage teamwork, support, and mutual understanding, making it possible for both partners to thrive.

6

Coping with Rejection Sensitivity

Rejection Sensitivity Dysphoria (RSD) is a term often used to describe the intense emotional response many individuals with ADHD experience when faced with perceived criticism, rejection, or failure. For women with ADHD, RSD can make even minor comments or situations feel deeply personal and overwhelming. In relationships, this sensitivity can lead to overreacting, withdrawing, or misinterpreting a partner's intentions.

Learning to manage RSD is essential for creating healthy relationships. By developing tools to navigate rejection sensitivity, women with ADHD can respond to perceived criticism with greater resilience and communicate their feelings in ways that build connection rather than conflict.

Understanding Rejection Sensitivity in ADHD

1. What is Rejection Sensitivity Dysphoria?

RSD occurs when individuals feel emotional pain from rejection or criticism more intensely than others might. It can be triggered by both real and perceived instances of rejection, making even neutral comments feel like personal attacks.

2. Common Triggers in Relationships

- Feeling criticized by a partner, even unintentionally.
- Perceiving indifference or lack of attention as rejection.
- Experiencing disagreements or feedback as personal failure.
- Comparing oneself to others and feeling inadequate.

3. How RSD Impacts Relationships

Women with RSD may react defensively or emotionally, escalating minor disagreements into major conflicts.

A fear of rejection can lead to people-pleasing or avoiding confrontation, which may cause resentment to build.

RSD can create a cycle of insecurity and overcompensation, leaving both partners feeling disconnected.

By understanding how RSD manifests, women with ADHD and their partners can approach these situations with empathy and strategies to reduce emotional intensity.

Zoe's Journey: Learning to Manage RSD in Her Relationship

Zoe, a 27-year-old with ADHD, often felt devastated by even small criticisms from her partner, Sam. If he pointed out that she'd forgotten a task or suggested a different way to do something, Zoe immediately felt like a failure. Her initial reaction was to withdraw, avoiding conversations for hours or even days. This pattern left both Zoe and Sam feeling frustrated and distant.

When Zoe learned about RSD as part of her ADHD diagnosis, she began to understand why her emotional responses felt so overwhelming. With guidance, she implemented strategies to manage her sensitivity and communicate her needs more effectively. Over time, these changes improved both her emotional well-being and her relationship.

Practical Strategies for Coping with RSD

1. Reframe Criticism as Constructive Feedback

Rather than viewing criticism as a personal attack, try to see it as information that can help you grow. Acknowledge that feedback isn't always about you as a person but about a specific behavior or situation.

Example: When Sam pointed out that Zoe had forgotten to pay a bill, Zoe reminded herself that this wasn't a comment on her worth but a practical observation. She thanked him for the reminder and set up an alert to avoid forgetting next time.

2. Ask for Clarification When Unsure

If a partner's comment feels hurtful, ask for clarification before reacting. Misunderstandings are common, and seeking clarification can prevent unnecessary conflict.

Example: When Sam said, "I feel like we're not on the same page this week," Zoe initially felt blamed. Instead of withdrawing, she asked, "What do you mean by that?" Sam explained that he felt disconnected, which opened the door for a productive conversation.

3. Practice Self-Soothing Techniques

When emotions start to escalate, use self-soothing strategies to calm your nervous system. Deep breathing, grounding exercises, or taking a brief walk can help you regain perspective before responding.

Example: Zoe developed a habit of stepping away for five minutes when she felt overwhelmed by criticism. During this time, she practiced deep breathing and reminded herself that she was loved and valued, regardless of her mistakes.

4. Create Scripts for Emotional Moments

Pre-planning how to respond to perceived criticism can help you avoid impulsive or defensive reactions. Simple phrases like "I need a moment to process that" or "Can we revisit this in a little while?" create space for reflection.

Example: When Sam suggested an alternative way to organize their shared schedule, Zoe initially felt criticized. Instead of reacting, she used her script: "That's an interesting idea. Let me think about it."

5. Focus on Positive Affirmations

Remind yourself of your strengths and contributions to the relationship. Positive affirmations can counterbalance the negative self-talk that often accompanies RSD.

Example: After a disagreement, Zoe would write affirmations like "I am learning and growing every day" or "I am loved and valued for who I am," which helped her regain emotional equilibrium.

Additional Strategies for Partners Supporting RSD

1. Use Gentle, Specific Language

Frame feedback in a way that feels constructive rather than critical. For example, instead of saying, "You always forget things," try, "It would help me if we set a reminder together for this task."

2. Acknowledge Emotional Reactions Without Judgment

Validate your partner's feelings without minimizing them. Statements like "I can see this feels really hard for you" show empathy and create a sense of safety.

3. Reassure Your Partner of Your Support

RSD often stems from a fear of rejection, so providing reassurance can help. Remind your partner that you care about them and are working together to build a strong relationship.

4. Be Patient and Avoid Escalating

Understand that managing RSD takes time and practice. If your partner reacts strongly, give them space to process their emotions rather than responding defensively.

Case Study: How Zoe and Sam Rebuilt Emotional Security

After learning about RSD, Zoe and Sam implemented a few key changes in their relationship. Sam made an effort to frame feedback constructively, using positive language and reassurance. Zoe practiced self-soothing techniques and clarified comments she found hurtful rather than assuming the worst.

For example, when Sam said, "You didn't lock the door when you left," Zoe's initial reaction was guilt and defensiveness. But instead of withdrawing, she paused and said, "I'm sorry about that. Thank you for catching it—I'll double-check next time." This response defused the tension and showed Sam that Zoe was actively working on managing her sensitivity.

Over time, these strategies helped Zoe feel more secure in her relationship. She stopped interpreting every comment as rejection, and Sam appreciated her openness to feedback. Together, they built a dynamic of mutual understanding and support.

Embracing RSD as Part of the Journey

Managing rejection sensitivity doesn't mean eliminating it entirely—it's about developing tools to navigate it with resilience and grace. By reframing criticism, practicing self-soothing, and communicating openly, women with ADHD can reduce the emotional intensity of RSD and strengthen their relationships.

Zoe's journey highlights the importance of self-awareness and collaboration. With effort and patience, RSD became less of a barrier and more of an opportunity for growth in her relationship. By fostering empathy, practicing self-compassion, and supporting one another, women with ADHD and their partners can create relationships that thrive on trust and understanding.

7

Time Management and Being Present in Relationships

For women with ADHD, managing time effectively and being fully present in relationships can feel like a balancing act. The challenges of ADHD—difficulty focusing, managing schedules, and transitioning between tasks—often interfere with the ability to prioritize quality time with a partner. However, developing time management strategies and practicing presence can foster deeper emotional connections and help women with ADHD create balance in their relationships.

Leah, a 30-year-old graphic designer with ADHD, often felt torn between her demanding job, personal projects, and her relationship. She loved her partner deeply but struggled to find enough energy and focus to fully engage during their time together. Leah's partner occasionally felt neglected, leading to conflicts that added to her feelings of guilt and inadequacy. Over time, Leah adopted practical strategies to manage her time better and stay present, transforming her relationship dynamics.

Understanding ADHD and Time Management Challenges

1. Time Blindness

Women with ADHD often struggle with time blindness, a difficulty in perceiving how much time tasks take or when they should start. This can lead to running late, missed appointments, or not allocating enough time for quality moments with a partner.

2. Hyper-Focus on Tasks or Projects

While hyper-focus can be a strength, it may result in losing track of time or neglecting other priorities. For example, a creative project or work assignment may inadvertently overshadow planned time with a partner.

3. Struggles with Transitions

Shifting attention from one task to another can be particularly challenging. For women with ADHD, transitioning from "work mode" to "relationship mode" often requires conscious effort and strategies to ensure they are fully present.

4. Overwhelm and Emotional Fatigue

Juggling multiple responsibilities can feel overwhelming, leading to emotional exhaustion. This can make it difficult to be emotionally available in a relationship, even when the intention is there.

45

By understanding these challenges, women with ADHD can develop strategies to manage time more effectively and ensure they're able to show up for their partners in meaningful ways.

Practical Time Management Strategies

1. Prioritize Quality Over Quantity

It's not always about how much time you spend with your partner but how present and engaged you are during that time. Scheduling short, uninterrupted periods of connection can have a significant impact. Even 15−20 minutes of focused attention can strengthen emotional bonds.

Example: Leah and her partner set aside 30 minutes each evening to talk about their day without distractions. This intentional time became a daily ritual that reinforced their connection.

2. Use Alarms, Timers, and Visual Cues

Setting reminders or alarms helps women with ADHD transition between tasks and avoid hyper-focusing for too long. Visual cues, such as a written schedule or sticky notes, can also serve as gentle prompts.

Example: Leah used a phone alarm to remind her when it was time to stop working and transition to dinner with her partner. This helped her maintain a balance between her career and personal life.

3. Create a Shared Calendar

Using a shared calendar can help couples align their schedules and set aside specific times for connection. This reduces the likelihood of missed plans and provides a clear structure for balancing responsibilities.

Example: Leah and her partner used a digital calendar to plan date nights, ensuring they both prioritized their time together.

4. Practice the "Two-Minute Rule"

For quick tasks, such as responding to a partner's text or tidying up a shared space, adopt the two-minute rule: If a task takes less than two minutes, do it immediately. This prevents small tasks from piling up and overwhelming the schedule.

Example: Leah made it a habit to immediately respond to her partner's important texts rather than letting them linger, which improved their communication.

5. Set Boundaries Around Work and Technology

Establishing boundaries for work hours and screen time helps prevent distractions during quality time. Turning off notifications, setting a phone on "Do Not Disturb," or physically removing devices can enhance focus and presence.

Example: Leah and her partner agreed to a "no phones at dinner" rule, allowing them to connect without interruptions.

Practical Tips for Being Fully Present

1. Practice Mindfulness to Ground Yourself

Engage in mindfulness techniques, such as deep breathing or focusing on sensory details, to center yourself in the moment. This can help shift attention from racing thoughts to your partner.

Example: Before sitting down for a conversation with her partner, Leah took three deep breaths to transition her focus from work to their time together.

2. Engage in Shared Activities

Doing activities together, like cooking, walking, or playing a game, helps create natural opportunities for connection and keeps both partners engaged.

Example: Leah and her partner started cooking dinner together once a week, turning it into a fun, collaborative activity that strengthened their bond.

3. Use Active Listening Techniques

Show your partner you're fully engaged by maintaining eye contact, nodding, and summarizing what they've said. Avoid interrupting or multitasking during conversations.

Example: When Leah's partner shared a story about his day, she made an effort to put down her phone, maintain eye contact, and ask follow-up questions.

4. Acknowledge and Redirect Wandering Attention

If you notice your mind wandering during a conversation, gently bring it back to the present moment without judgment. A simple mental note like "Come back to now" can help.

Example: Leah found herself drifting during a discussion, so she refocused by repeating her partner's last sentence to herself.

Case Study: Leah's Journey to Balancing Time and Presence

Leah's partner had expressed frustration about her frequent distraction and tendency to work late into the night. Recognizing the strain this placed on their relationship, Leah implemented small but meaningful changes. She set an alarm each evening to remind herself to stop working, established a shared calendar with her partner, and practiced mindfulness techniques to stay present during conversations.

One of the most impactful changes Leah made was dedicating Saturday mornings as "quality time" with her partner. During this time, they went for walks, tried new breakfast recipes, or simply talked. These intentional efforts helped Leah balance her responsibilities while showing her partner that she valued their time together.

Over time, Leah's partner noticed and appreciated her efforts. Their conflicts decreased, and they both felt more connected and aligned in their relationship.

Additional Tips for Partners Supporting ADHD Time Challenges

1. Provide Gentle Reminders

If your partner tends to lose track of time, offer reminders in a supportive way. For example, "We have dinner in 15 minutes— let's wrap up what you're doing."

2. Be Flexible and Adaptable

Recognize that time management is a work in progress for women with ADHD. Offering patience and understanding can reduce stress and help your partner feel supported.

3. Appreciate the Efforts

Acknowledge and celebrate even small changes in time management or presence. Statements like, "I noticed you stopped working on time today, and I really appreciate it," reinforce positive habits.

Embracing Balance and Presence in Relationships

Balancing responsibilities while being present in a relationship requires effort, especially for women with ADHD. By prioritizing quality time, practicing mindfulness, and using tools like shared calendars and timers, women can manage their time effectively and foster deeper emotional connections with their partners.

Leah's journey shows that small, consistent changes can make a big difference. With patience, intention, and communication, women with ADHD can create relationships where both partners feel valued, understood, and deeply connected.

8

Developing a Support System

For women with ADHD, having a strong support system beyond a romantic relationship is essential. A diverse network of friends, family, and peers provides emotional support, practical advice, and a sense of community that eases the pressure on a primary relationship. Developing a support system can also help women feel understood and validated in ways that enhance their confidence and overall well-being.

Kim, a 36-year-old social worker with ADHD, often relied solely on her partner, Mark, for emotional support. While Mark was understanding, Kim's dependency on him for validation and problem-solving sometimes left him feeling overwhelmed. Recognizing the need for a broader network, Kim began cultivating a support system that included friends, family, and ADHD-specific communities. This shift not only strengthened her relationship with Mark but also improved her overall resilience and self-esteem.

The Importance of a Support System for Women with ADHD

1. Reducing Pressure on the Primary Relationship

Relying solely on a romantic partner for emotional or logistical support can strain the relationship. A strong network provides additional outlets for advice, empathy, and shared experiences, creating a more balanced dynamic.

2. Fostering Connection and Understanding

Engaging with others who share similar challenges, such as ADHD-specific support groups, can provide a sense of belonging and validation. This reduces feelings of isolation and promotes self-acceptance.

3. Gaining Practical Insights

A diverse support system offers a variety of perspectives and advice. For example, friends with ADHD may share strategies for managing symptoms, while family members might provide practical assistance during stressful times.

4. Enhancing Self-Esteem and Independence

Feeling connected to a broader community reinforces self-worth and encourages women to take initiative in managing their challenges. This independence empowers them to bring their best selves to their romantic relationships.

Practical Steps to Build a Support System

1. Reconnect with Trusted Friends and Family

Reaching out to supportive individuals from your existing circle can strengthen bonds and create a reliable safety net. Start with small gestures, like sending a thoughtful message or scheduling a coffee date.

Example: Kim rekindled her friendship with an old college roommate, who became a valuable source of emotional support and laughter during stressful times.

2. Join ADHD-Specific Communities

Online forums, social media groups, or local meetups for women with ADHD offer a space to share experiences, exchange tips, and feel understood. These communities provide validation and practical advice tailored to ADHD-related challenges.

Example: Kim joined an online group for women with ADHD, where she discovered helpful time management strategies and formed friendships with others who shared her experiences.

3. Engage in Shared Activities

Participating in group activities, like hobbies, classes, or volunteer work, creates opportunities to connect with like-minded individuals. These settings often lead to organic friendships and a sense of purpose.

Example: Kim started attending a weekly yoga class, where she bonded with others who valued mindfulness and self-care.

4. Seek Professional Support When Needed

Therapists, coaches, and ADHD specialists offer targeted guidance and tools to navigate challenges. Regular sessions can provide a safe space for processing emotions and building skills.

Example: Kim worked with a therapist to improve her emotional regulation and communication skills, which enhanced her relationships both inside and outside her support system.

5. Set Boundaries and Manage Expectations

While building connections, it's essential to establish healthy boundaries. Avoid over-relying on any one person, and ensure relationships are mutually supportive.

Example: Kim maintained a balance by checking in with her support network regularly but also respecting their time and boundaries.

Case Study: Kim's Journey in Expanding Her Support System

Before building her support system, Kim leaned heavily on Mark for emotional reassurance, which sometimes led to feelings of guilt and frustration on both sides. After reflecting on the dynamic, Kim decided to expand her network.

Steps Kim Took to Build Her Support System:

1. Reaching Out to Old Friends: Kim started reconnecting with friends by sending short, friendly messages. She focused on rebuilding trust and gradually deepened these relationships.

2. Exploring ADHD Communities: Kim joined a local ADHD meetup group, where she learned effective strategies for managing her symptoms and found camaraderie with others who understood her challenges.

3. Seeking Professional Guidance: Kim scheduled sessions with a therapist who helped her navigate rejection sensitivity and set realistic goals for her personal growth.

4. Balancing New Connections with Old Relationships: While nurturing her support system, Kim ensured that her relationship with Mark remained a priority. She communicated her progress and shared her experiences, which strengthened their connection.

Over time, Kim noticed a significant improvement in her emotional resilience. Having multiple sources of support allowed her to navigate challenges with confidence, and her relationship with Mark became less strained as she gained independence and self-assurance.

DEVELOPING A SUPPORT SYSTEM

Practical Tips for Partners Supporting the Development of a Support System

1. Encourage Your Partner's Efforts

Celebrate their steps toward building connections, whether it's joining a group or reconnecting with a friend. Positive reinforcement builds confidence and shows your support.

2. Be Open to Sharing the Emotional Load

Understand that your partner may need additional sources of support to thrive. Encourage them to seek guidance from others when necessary.

3. Participate in Shared Activities

Join your partner in exploring new hobbies or community groups, fostering shared experiences while helping them expand their network.

4. Respect Their Independence

Allow your partner the space to develop their support system without feeling the need to be involved in every aspect. This encourages personal growth and autonomy.

Balancing Support Systems with Primary Relationships

While developing a support system, it's important to maintain balance and ensure that the primary relationship remains a priority. Open communication, regular check-ins, and intentional quality time help preserve emotional intimacy while fostering independence.

Kim and Mark found a routine that worked for them: Kim dedicated time each week to her friends and ADHD group, while also setting aside regular date nights with Mark. This balance allowed them to nurture both their individual growth and their connection as a couple.

Embracing Community as a Source of Strength

For women with ADHD, building a support system is not just a practical step—it's an act of self-care. Engaging with friends, family, and peers creates a sense of belonging and validation, empowering women to navigate challenges with confidence. When relationships are balanced with a broader network of support, they become healthier, more resilient, and more fulfilling.

Kim's journey demonstrates the transformative power of connection. By diversifying her support system, she found the strength and tools to thrive, while also deepening her relationship with Mark. A strong support system doesn't replace a romantic partner—it enhances the partnership by fostering independence, resilience, and mutual respect.

9

Strengthening Intimacy and Connection

Intimacy and connection are the cornerstones of a strong relationship, but for women with ADHD, certain traits—like distractibility, impulsivity, or emotional intensity—can sometimes complicate these aspects. On the flip side, ADHD also brings unique strengths, such as creativity, empathy, and spontaneity, which can deepen emotional and physical intimacy. By embracing these strengths and addressing the challenges with practical strategies, women with ADHD can foster a deeper connection with their partners.

Rachel, a 40-year-old artist with ADHD, loved her husband deeply but often felt that their emotional and physical connection had taken a backseat to their busy lives. Her ADHD made it difficult for her to focus during intimate moments, and she sometimes misinterpreted her husband's need for space as a lack of affection. Recognizing this, Rachel and her husband worked together to create intentional moments of connection, reigniting the spark in their relationship.

The Impact of ADHD on Intimacy

1. Distractibility During Intimate Moments

Women with ADHD may find their minds wandering during emotional or physical intimacy, which can leave their partner feeling disconnected or unimportant. This isn't a lack of interest but rather a symptom of ADHD that requires gentle redirection.

2. Emotional Sensitivity and Vulnerability

Emotional sensitivity can make women with ADHD hyper-aware of perceived changes in their partner's mood or affection, sometimes leading to overthinking or feelings of insecurity.

3. Hyper-Focus on Challenges

When ADHD leads to hyper-focus on unresolved conflicts or personal stress, it can be difficult to fully engage in the present moment, which may impact intimacy.

4. Strengths That Enhance Intimacy

On the positive side, women with ADHD are often deeply empathetic, creative, and spontaneous, which can bring excitement, playfulness, and depth to their relationships.

By understanding these dynamics, women with ADHD can embrace their strengths while addressing the challenges to create a more balanced and fulfilling intimate connection.

Practical Strategies for Strengthening Intimacy

1. Create Intentional Intimacy Rituals

Set aside regular, intentional time for emotional and physical intimacy. This could include weekly date nights, morning cuddles, or quiet evenings spent talking without distractions. Consistency helps create a safe space for connection.

Example: Rachel and her husband established Friday nights as their "connection time," where they turned off their phones, lit candles, and spent the evening talking and reconnecting.

2. Communicate Needs and Preferences Openly

Talk openly with your partner about your emotional and physical needs, as well as any ADHD-related challenges that might impact intimacy. Clear communication fosters understanding and helps both partners feel heard.

Example: Rachel explained to her husband that she sometimes struggled to focus during conversations and asked him to gently redirect her attention when necessary.

3. Use Sensory Grounding During Intimate Moments

Ground yourself in the present moment by focusing on sensory details, such as touch, sound, or smell. This helps redirect attention away from wandering thoughts and back to your partner.

Example: During a quiet moment with her husband, Rachel focused on the sound of his voice and the feeling of his hand in hers, which helped her stay present and connected.

4. Explore Love Languages

Understanding and expressing love through your partner's preferred love language—whether it's acts of service, words of affirmation, quality time, physical touch, or gifts—can deepen intimacy and connection.

Example: Rachel's husband valued words of affirmation, so she made an effort to write him thoughtful notes or verbally express her appreciation, which strengthened their bond.

5. Incorporate Playfulness and Creativity

Embrace the spontaneity and creativity that ADHD often brings. Plan playful surprises, try new activities together, or find ways to inject humor into your relationship to keep things fresh and exciting.

Example: Rachel surprised her husband with a spontaneous painting session in their backyard, turning an ordinary evening into a memorable experience.

6. Address Emotional Barriers

If unresolved conflicts or personal insecurities are creating distance, take time to address these issues through open communication, therapy, or self-reflection. Emotional clarity lays the foundation for deeper intimacy.

Example: Rachel and her husband scheduled regular check-ins to discuss any lingering issues, which helped them clear emotional barriers and feel closer.

Practical Tips for Physical Intimacy

1. Focus on Small Gestures

Physical intimacy doesn't always have to involve grand gestures. Small actions, like holding hands, hugging, or sharing a kiss, create a sense of closeness and reinforce emotional connection.

Example: Rachel made it a habit to hug her husband every morning before they started their day, which became a simple yet meaningful ritual.

2. Reduce Distractions During Intimate Moments

Turn off phones, dim the lights, and create an environment that minimizes distractions. This helps both partners feel fully present and connected.

Example: Rachel and her husband designated their bedroom as a "no-screen zone" during evenings, which helped them focus on each other without outside interruptions.

3. Practice Mindful Touch

Slow down and pay attention to physical sensations during intimate moments. This not only helps with focus but also enhances the emotional connection between partners.

Example: Rachel practiced mindful touch by focusing on the feeling of her husband's embrace, which deepened their physical connection.

4. Communicate Preferences with Kindness

If certain ADHD traits, like distractibility or sensory sensitivities, impact physical intimacy, discuss them openly with your partner and explore alternatives that work for both of you.

Example: Rachel explained to her husband that certain fabrics irritated her skin, so they adjusted their bedding to create a more comfortable environment.

Case Study: Rachel's Journey to Intentional Intimacy

Before prioritizing intimacy, Rachel and her husband often felt disconnected due to their busy schedules and ADHD-related challenges. Rachel's tendency to zone out during conversations sometimes made her husband feel unimportant, while her sensitivity to perceived criticism created emotional barriers.

Through intentional efforts, Rachel and her husband rebuilt their connection. They established weekly rituals, openly discussed their needs, and incorporated playful activities into their routine. These changes not only strengthened their physical and emotional intimacy but also brought a renewed sense of joy and partnership to their relationship.

Key Changes Rachel Implemented:

1. Set a Weekly Date Night: Friday evenings became their dedicated time for connection.

2. Communicated Love Through Words: Rachel expressed her appreciation through notes and affirmations.

3. Focused on Sensory Details: Mindfulness helped Rachel stay present during intimate moments.

4. Explored New Experiences Together: Playful activities, like impromptu art sessions, brought excitement back into their relationship.

Over time, Rachel and her husband found that their relationship felt stronger and more fulfilling than ever.

Embracing Intimacy as a Journey

Strengthening intimacy in a relationship isn't about achieving perfection—it's about showing up for each other with empathy, intention, and love. For women with ADHD, embracing their unique strengths and addressing challenges with curiosity and compassion can lead to a deeper and more authentic connection.

Rachel's journey shows that intimacy is an ongoing process, built through small, intentional acts and open communication. By prioritizing emotional and physical connection, women with ADHD can create relationships that are not only resilient but also deeply fulfilling.

10

Creating a Relationship Growth Plan

Healthy relationships don't just happen—they require effort, intention, and a shared commitment to growth. For women with ADHD, a structured approach to nurturing a relationship can be incredibly beneficial. A relationship growth plan serves as a roadmap for identifying areas of improvement, celebrating successes, and ensuring both partners feel valued and supported.

Beth, a 38-year-old lawyer with ADHD, often felt overwhelmed by the day-to-day demands of her relationship. She and her partner, James, loved each other deeply, but they sometimes struggled with communication and balancing responsibilities. Realizing the importance of intentional growth, Beth and James developed a relationship growth plan that helped them address challenges, set goals, and build a stronger partnership over time.

What is a Relationship Growth Plan?

A relationship growth plan is a structured framework for couples to set goals, track progress, and regularly evaluate the health of their relationship. It's not about perfection or rigid rules but about fostering intentionality and accountability. For women with ADHD, this plan can provide clarity, structure, and a sense of accomplishment, helping to reduce feelings of overwhelm.

Key elements of a relationship growth plan include:

1. Identifying Strengths and Challenges

Acknowledging what's working well in the relationship and areas that need improvement.

2. Setting Relationship Goals

Creating short-term and long-term goals that align with the couple's values and priorities.

3. Establishing Check-In Rituals

Scheduling regular times to discuss progress, celebrate successes, and address concerns.

4. Adapting the Plan Over Time

Remaining flexible and adjusting the plan as the relationship evolves.

Practical Steps to Create a Relationship Growth Plan

1. Reflect on the Current State of the Relationship

Start by discussing the current strengths and challenges of the relationship. Focus on what each partner appreciates and what they'd like to work on.

Example: Beth and James identified communication as an area for improvement and recognized their shared love of travel as a strength they wanted to nurture.

2. Set SMART Goals

Goals should be Specific, Measurable, Achievable, Relevant, and Time-bound. For example, instead of saying, "We want to communicate better," a SMART goal would be, "We will have weekly check-ins every Sunday to discuss any concerns."

Example: Beth and James set a goal to dedicate 30 minutes each evening to uninterrupted quality time, free from phones or other distractions.

3. Develop Actionable Steps for Each Goal

Break down each goal into smaller, actionable steps. This makes goals feel more achievable and provides clear direction.

Example: To improve communication, Beth and James agreed to practice active listening techniques during conversations and use "I" statements to express their feelings.

4. Schedule Regular Check-Ins

Set aside time to review the plan together. Use these check-ins to evaluate progress, celebrate wins, and adjust the plan as needed. Monthly or biweekly check-ins work well for most couples.

Example: On the last Sunday of each month, Beth and James reviewed their goals, shared feedback, and planned for the month ahead.

5. Celebrate Milestones and Achievements

Acknowledge and celebrate progress, no matter how small. This reinforces positive behaviors and keeps both partners motivated.

Example: After three months of consistent check-ins, Beth and James celebrated their progress with a weekend getaway.

6. Adapt to Changing Needs

Relationships evolve, and so should the growth plan. Be open to revising goals and strategies as circumstances change.

Example: When Beth started a new job with longer hours, she

and James adjusted their plan to include shorter, more frequent check-ins.

Case Study: Beth and James' Journey with a Relationship Growth Plan

Before implementing their growth plan, Beth and James often felt like they were "winging it" in their relationship. Conflicts sometimes lingered unresolved, and busy schedules left little time for meaningful connection. Creating a structured plan helped them approach their relationship with intention and focus.

Steps Beth and James Took:

1. Identified Priorities: They agreed that improving communication and spending more quality time together were their top priorities.

2. Set Goals: They established clear goals, such as having weekly check-ins and planning a monthly date night.

3. Tracked Progress: During their monthly reviews, they reflected on what was working and what needed adjustment.

4. Celebrated Wins: They acknowledged each other's efforts, which deepened their appreciation and reinforced positive

habits.

Over time, Beth and James noticed significant improvements in their relationship. They argued less, felt more connected, and developed a deeper sense of partnership. The growth plan provided a framework that kept them aligned and focused on nurturing their bond.

Additional Tips for Building a Growth Plan

1. Focus on Collaboration

A growth plan is a joint effort. Ensure both partners have an equal voice in setting goals and creating action steps.

2. Be Realistic and Flexible

Avoid overloading the plan with too many goals at once. Focus on one or two priorities at a time and adjust as needed.

3. Use Tools for Organization

Consider using shared tools, like a digital calendar or a relationship journal, to keep track of goals and progress.

4. Balance Structure with Spontaneity

While structure is important, leave room for spontaneity and playfulness in the relationship. This keeps things fresh and prevents the plan from feeling too rigid.

How Partners Can Support the Process

1. Encourage Open Dialogue

Create a safe space for your partner to share their thoughts, goals, and concerns without fear of judgment.

2. Show Appreciation for Efforts

Recognize the effort your partner puts into the growth plan, even if progress feels slow.

3. Be Patient with Setbacks

Growth isn't linear. If challenges arise, approach them with patience and a willingness to adapt.

4. Stay Committed to the Process

Consistency is key. Regularly revisit the plan to ensure it remains a priority for both partners.

Embracing Growth as a Journey

Creating and maintaining a relationship growth plan is about building a partnership that evolves with intention and care. It's not about fixing flaws or achieving perfection but about fostering a dynamic that supports mutual understanding, respect, and love.

Beth and James' journey illustrates the power of a growth plan to transform a relationship. By setting goals, celebrating progress, and remaining flexible, they cultivated a connection that was both resilient and fulfilling. For women with ADHD, a structured plan provides clarity and direction, making it easier to navigate challenges and nurture the relationship.

As you embark on this journey, remember that growth is a continuous process. Celebrate the small wins, stay open to change, and trust in your ability to build a relationship that thrives on love, empathy, and shared purpose.